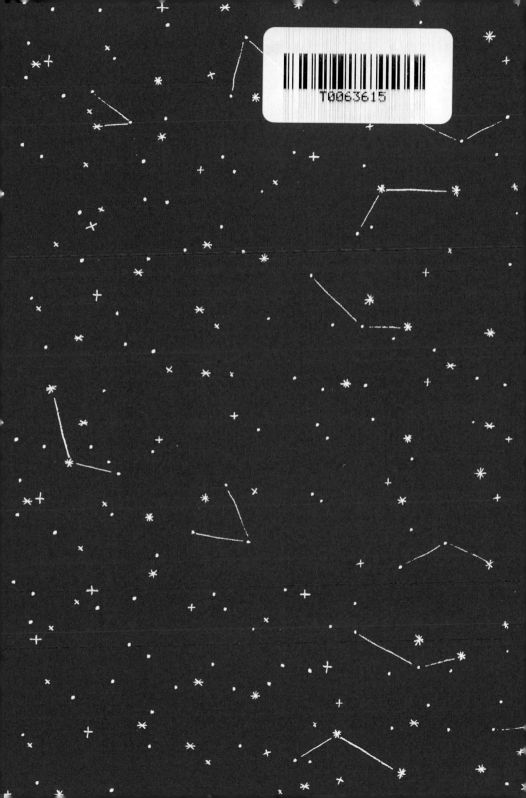

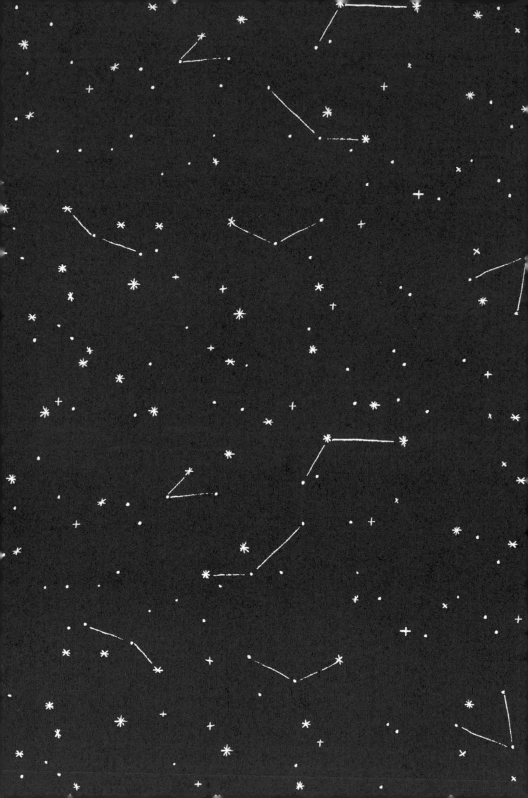

Bedtime Book for Bump

To Pippy

-R.S.

For my Mum and Dad, to the moon and back.

-A.B.

MAYO CLINIC PRESS
200 First St. SW
Rochester, MN 55905
MCPress.MayoClinic.org

To stay informed about Mayo Clinic Press, please subscribe to our free
e-newsletter at MCPress.MayoClinic.org/parenting or follow us on social media.

For bulk sales, contact Mayo Clinic at SpecialSalesMayoBooks@mayo.edu.

**Proceeds from the sale of every book benefit important medical research and
education at Mayo Clinic.**

First American Edition 2024

ISBN: 979-8-887-70185-1 (hardcover)

Library of Congress Cataloging-in-Publication Data is available upon request.
Printed and bound in China.

Bedtime Book for Bump

MAYO CLINIC PRESS KIDS

The benefits of reading to your bump

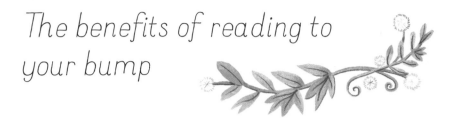

Congratulations! Waiting for a baby is such a special time. Months spent counting down until that moment when your baby is born and you finally meet the next little love of your life for the very first time. But birth isn't the beginning of it all. Your relationship with your baby begins before you even meet. Pregnancy is a truly miraculous time when your tiny human is already listening, learning, and even dreaming about the world around them. Babies in utero are developing at incredible rates. During the third trimester their brains are making over one million neural connections per second. Your baby is learning so much by sucking, tasting, touching, and listening to their birthing parent's body, as well as their own.

From around week 25 forward, the rhythmic sounds of your voices are soothing your baby—the sound of both parents' voices is so calming that it lowers your baby's heart rate. Your baby is getting to know you through the sound of your voices and will even learn to recognize your voices before they are born. Even within an hour of birth, newborns prefer the sound of their parents' voice to a stranger's voice and prefer to listen to a story that was read to them repeatedly while they were in the womb.

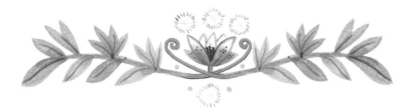

So, talking to your baby, singing to your baby, and reading to your baby during your pregnancy is not only an innate bonding experience, but it can also become a relaxing ritual for both parent and baby. As you read this beautiful poem aloud to your baby, their heart rate will slow as they listen, because your baby is falling in love with your voice and is calmed by the familiarity of the verse. There is so much comfort in the familiar—even for tiny babies.

And when you do meet your baby, the sound of your voice—the same voice that read this poem to them over and over again—will reassure them that, even though this new world is so very different from everything they knew before, they are already home, right there in your arms.

On the next page there's a space for you to write a letter to your baby before they are born and, after they are born, a page to dedicate this book to them and record their date of birth and their birth weight. At the back of the book you'll find an envelope, perfect for keeping baby scan photos and other precious mementos of your pregnancy.

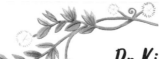

Dr. Kimberley Bennett

PsyD—Child, Adolescent, and Educational Psychology

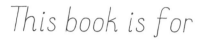

This book is for

. . . .

Born

. . . .

Weight

. . . .

Use this space to write a letter to
your baby before they are born

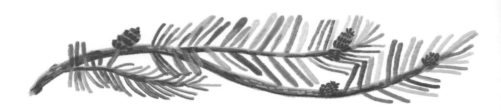

Little One, this book's for you,

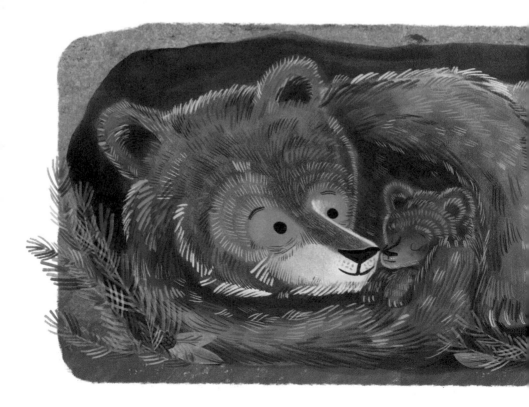

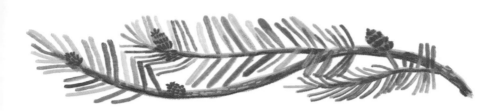

I'll read it loud and clear.

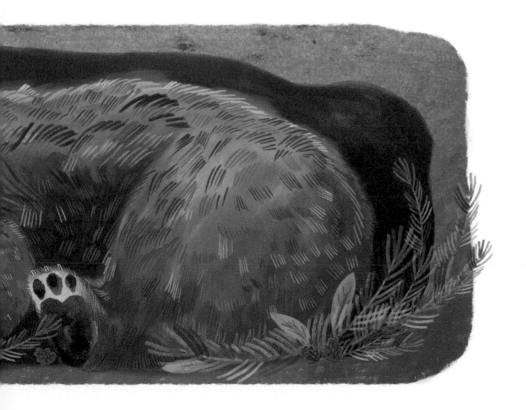

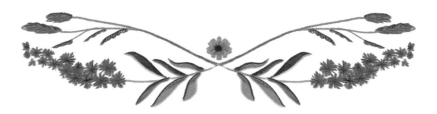

For though we
haven't met you yet,

I know that you can hear.

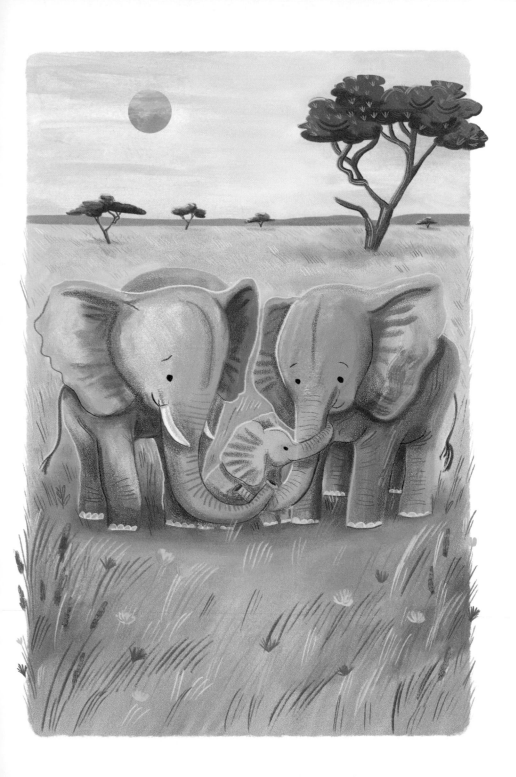

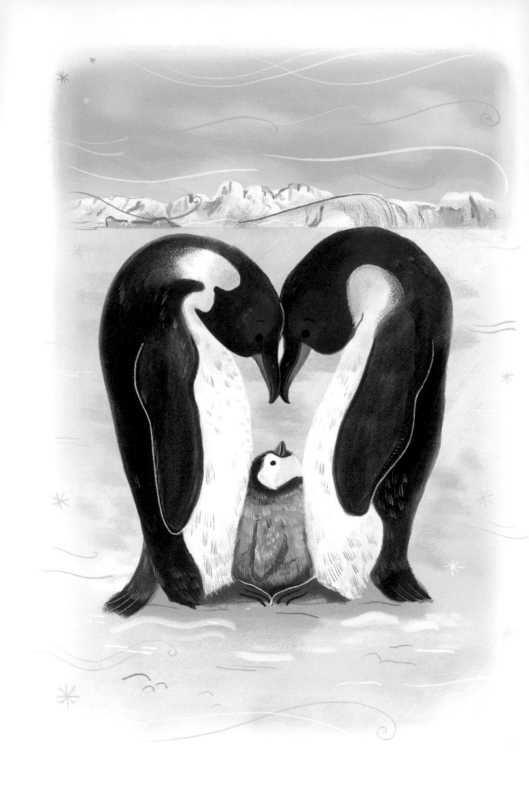

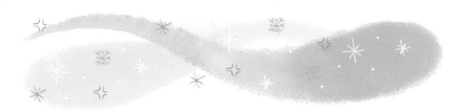

Your mother's beating heart

makes up the music
of your day,

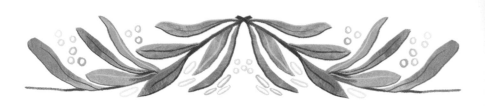

And when I sing,
you listen in:

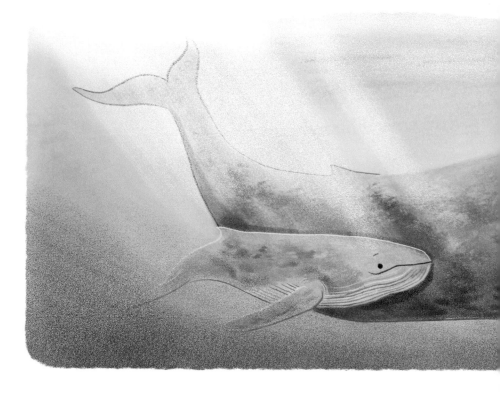

You wriggle and you play.

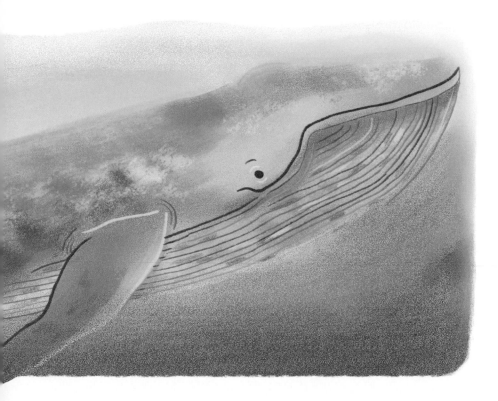

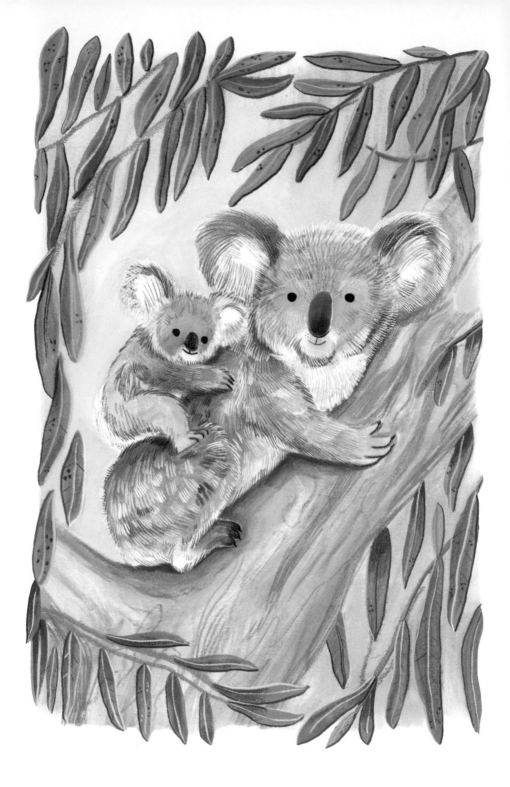

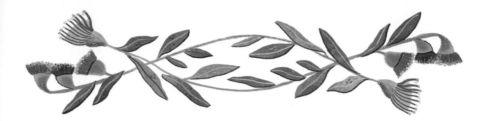

We've yet to hear
you laugh or cry;

We've yet to see your smile.

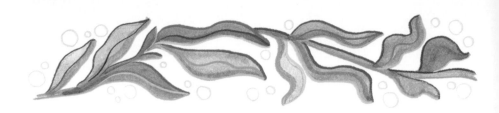

But you hear every
word we say,

so let's just talk a while...

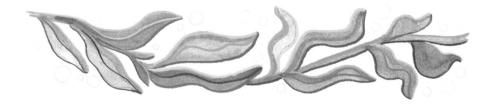

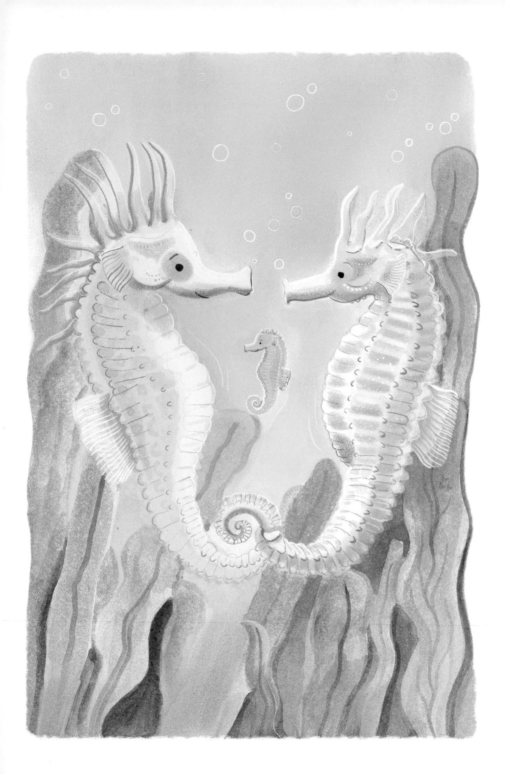

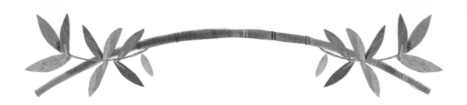

One day I'll read you stories,

when you're curled
inside my arms.

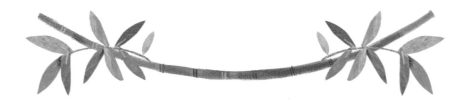

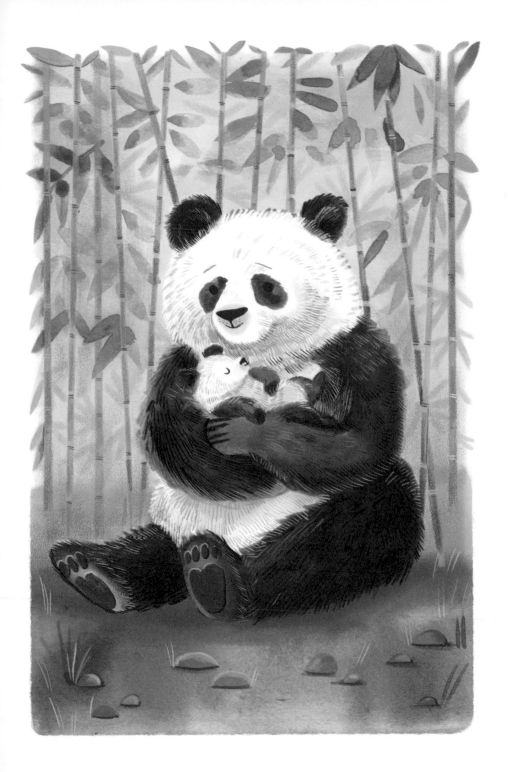

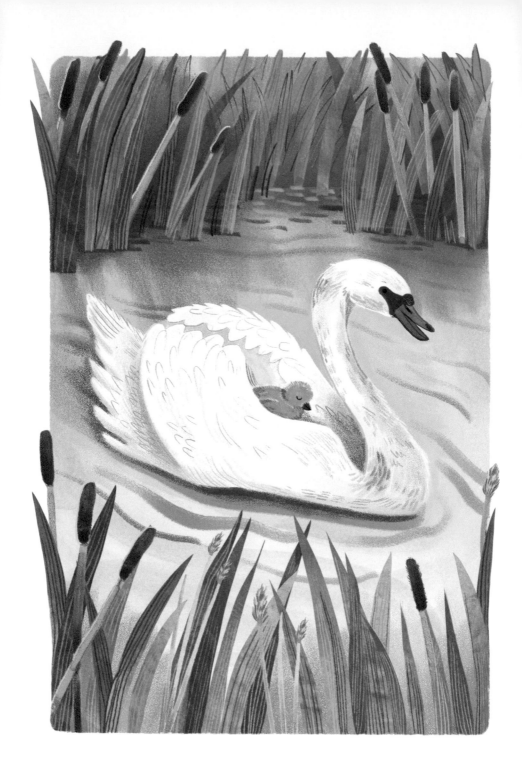

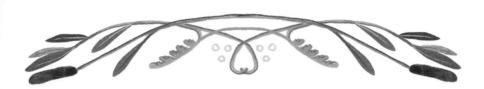

And the music of my words

will let you know
you're safe from harm.

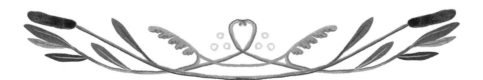

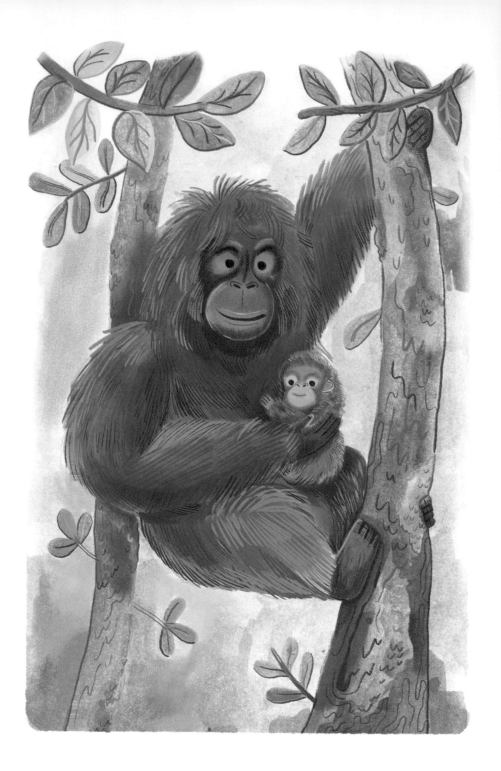

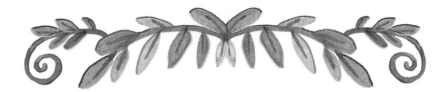

One day I'll show
you pictures,

while you're sitting on my knee,

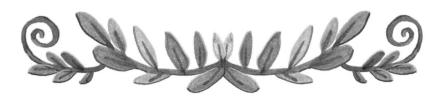

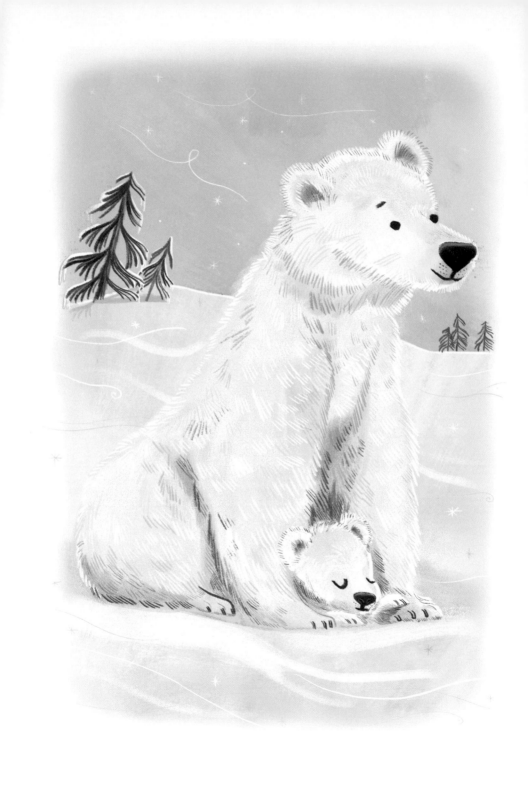

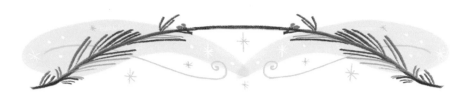

And I'll hold your
little hand so tight

as you lean into me.

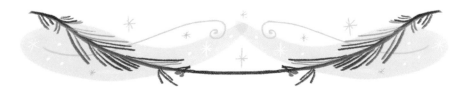

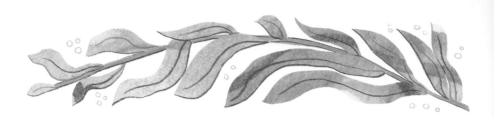

One day I'll rock
you as you sleep,

your head upon my chest.

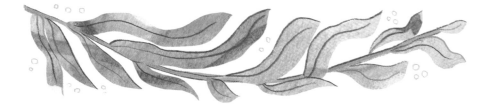

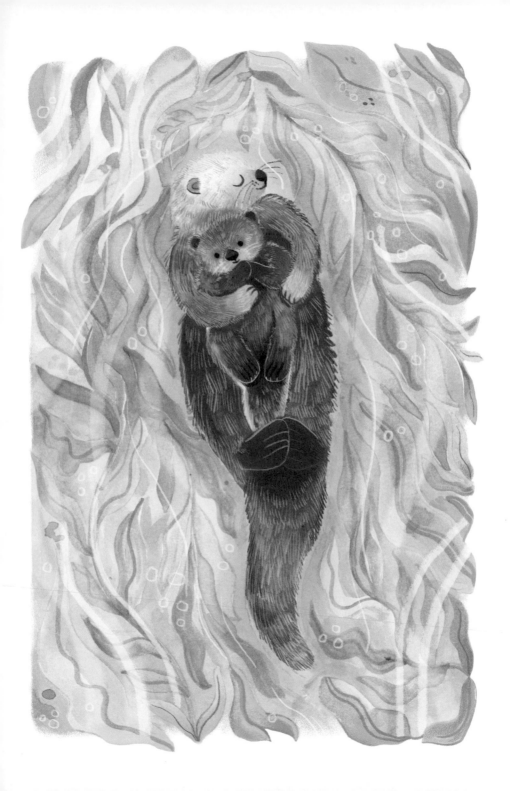

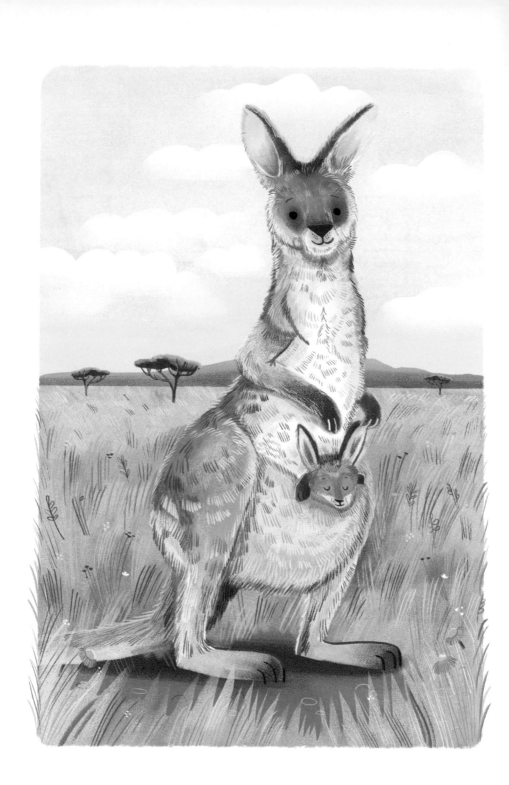

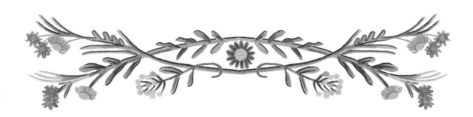

But now you're snuggled
in your bump –

the perfect place to rest.

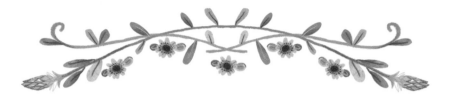

This book's for you,
our little one,

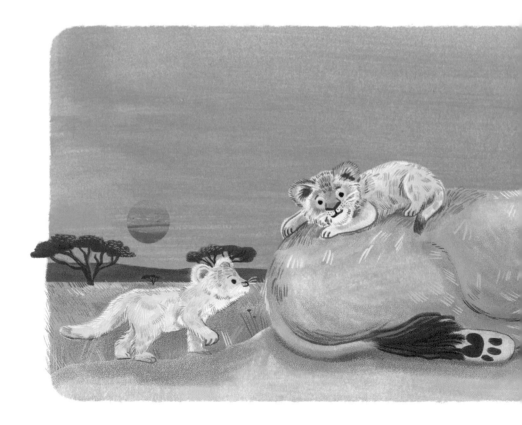

It's how our story starts.

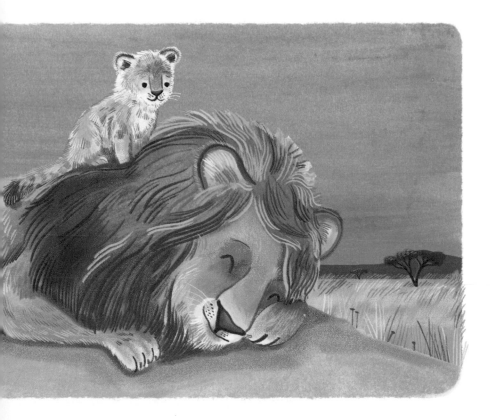

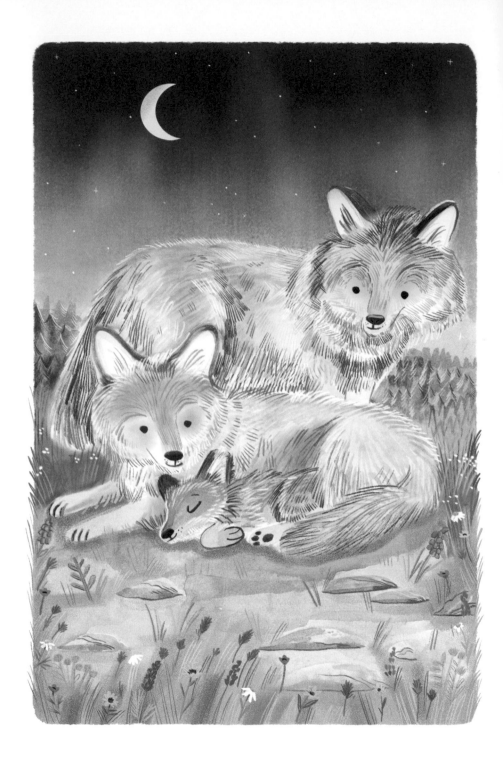

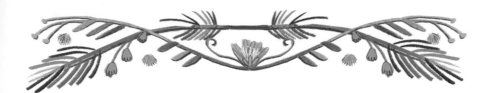

A promise that
I make to you,

with words that
speak my heart.

And when we see you
face to face,

and gaze into your eyes,

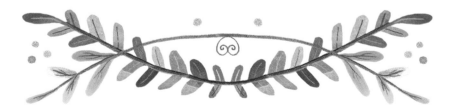

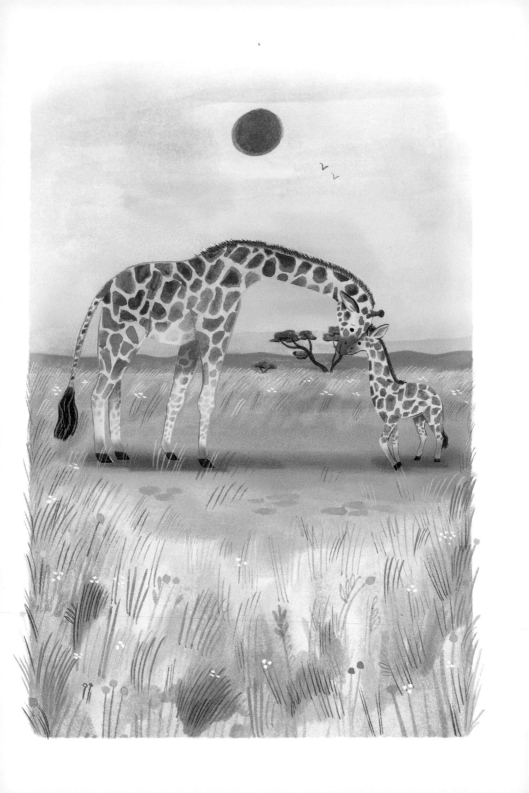

The world will be

so new to you—

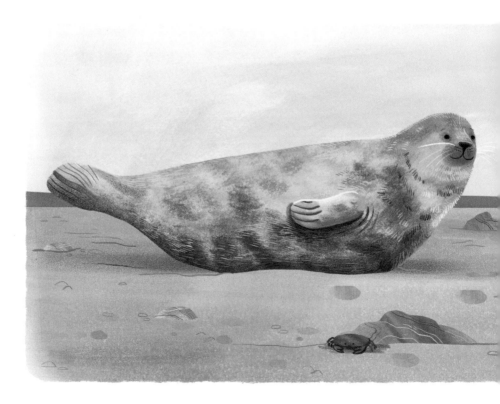

A marvelous surprise.

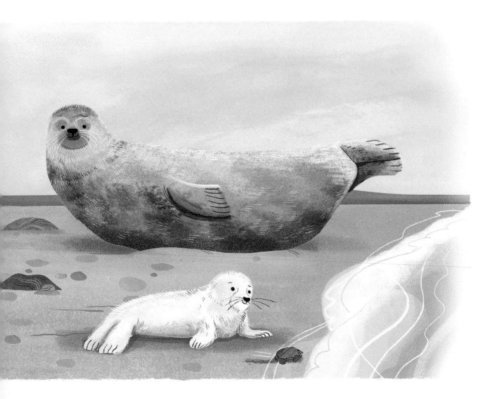

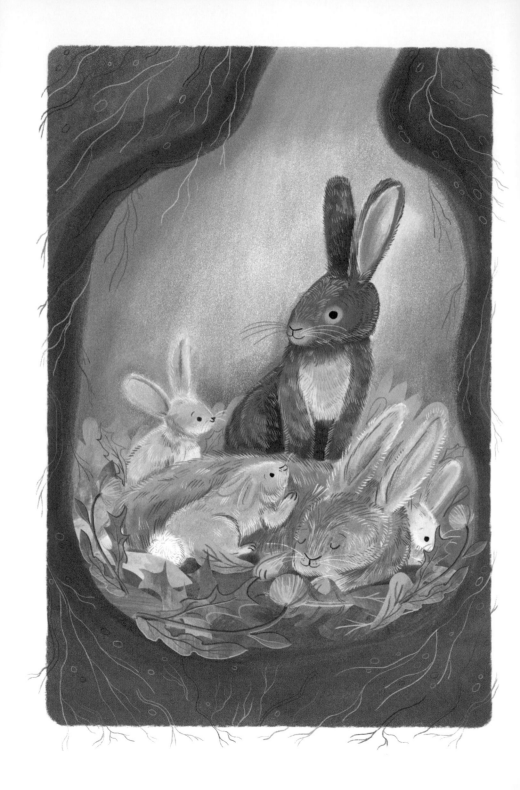

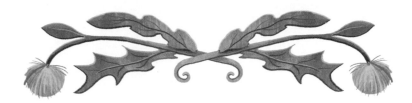

But one thing you'll
already know,

familiar and near,

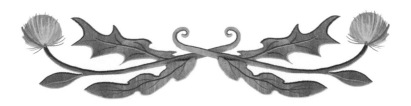

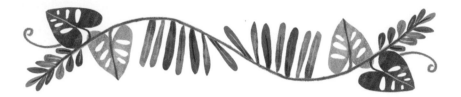

My voice will be here,
just the same,

to whisper in your ear.

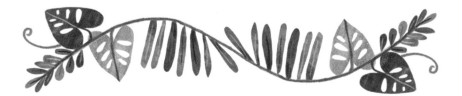

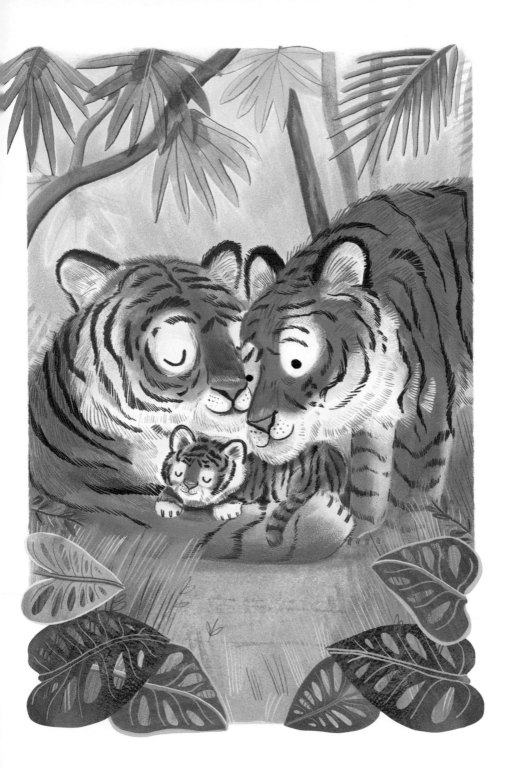

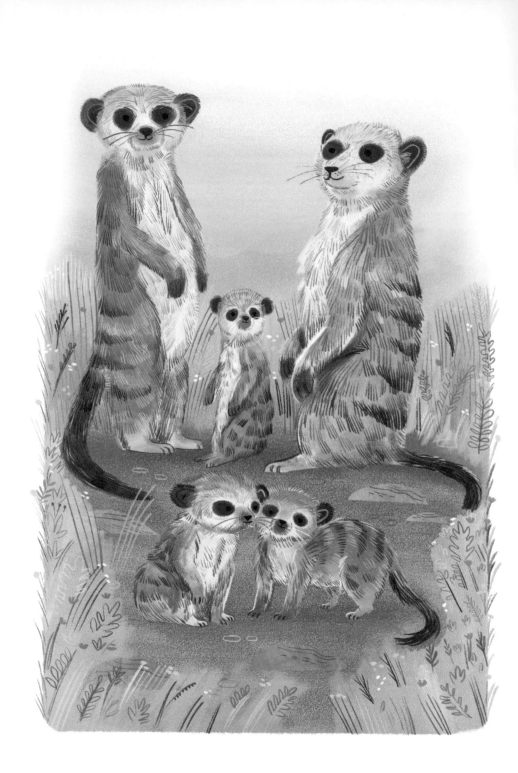

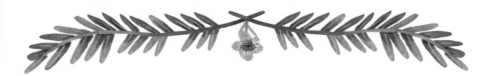

I'll tell you that you're
loved, and safe,

our very greatest treasure.

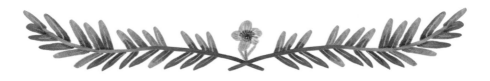

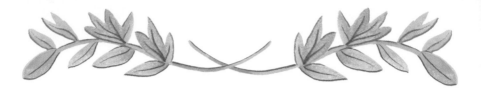

And my words will wrap
you in their love,

from now until forever.

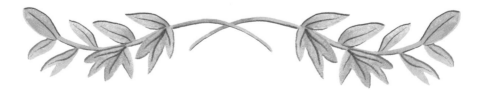

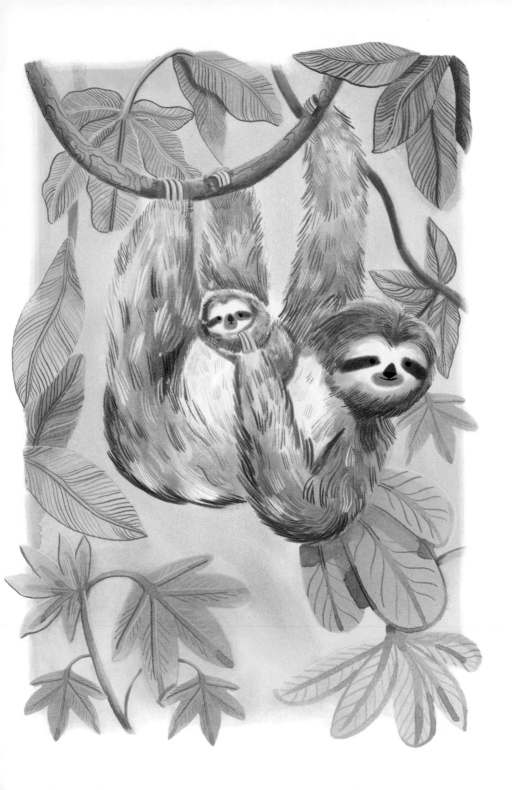

Use the envelope at the back of this book to keep your most treasured mementos of your pregnancy.

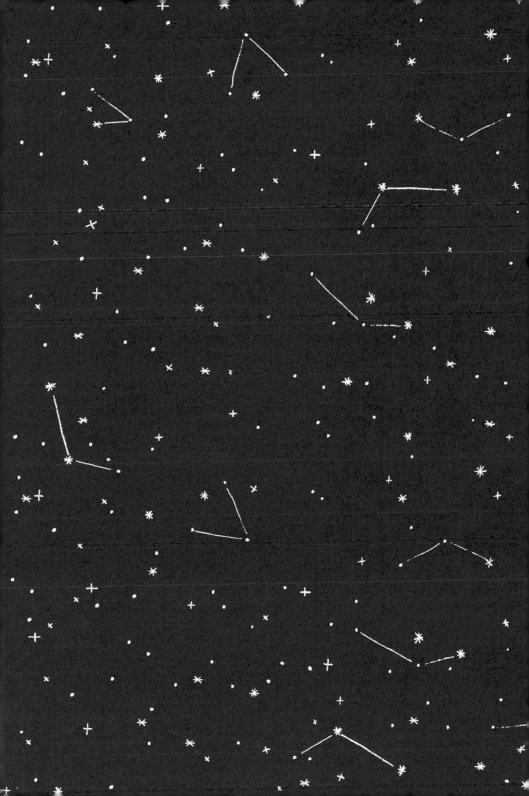

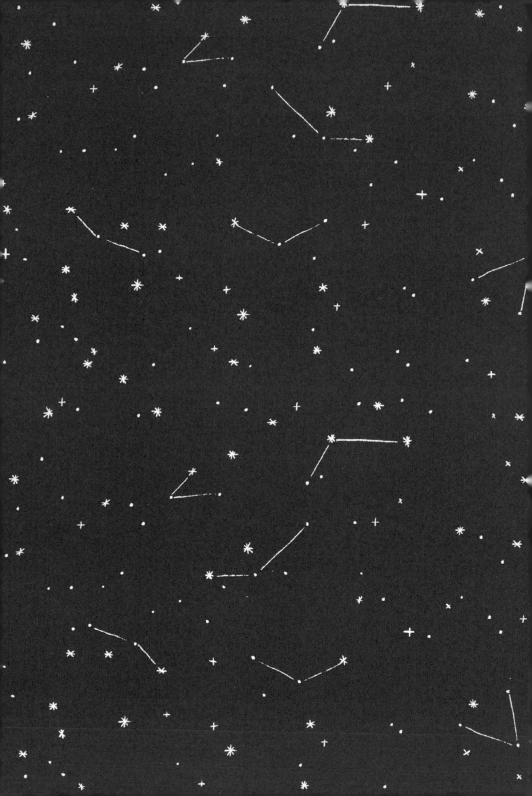